Balancing Blood Sugar:

A Comprehensive Guide to Diabetes Meal Planning and Nutritious Eating

By

Richard B. Peltier

DISCLAIMER

The material presented in this book, ***"Balancing Blood Sugar: A Comprehensive Guide to Diabetes Meal Planning and Nutritious Eating,"*** is meant for educational purposes only and should not be used in lieu of expert medical guidance, diagnosis, or treatment.. The material given here is based on general knowledge and suggestions known up to the publishing date, which is the extent of the model's knowledge cut-off (September 2022).

 Individuals with diabetes or any other health condition should always consult with qualified healthcare professionals, such as doctors, registered dieticians, certified diabetes educators, or other specialized healthcare providers, to receive personalized advice and recommendations tailored to their specific health needs and circumstances.

The writers and publishers of this book have taken reasonable measures to guarantee the accuracy and currency of the material given. However, they do not make any warranties or claims about the completeness, accuracy, reliability, or appropriateness of the material for any specific purpose.

The authors and publishers disclaim all responsibility for any bad effects or repercussions stemming from the use of the material contained herein.

Readers are recommended to use their discretion and judgment in applying the information presented in this book to their unique circumstances. Any reliance on the information presented in this book is totally at the reader's own risk.

Medical knowledge and standards about diabetes care and treatment may develop over time. Therefore, readers are recommended to keep themselves updated about the newest breakthroughs in diabetes research and contact healthcare specialists for the most up-to-date and relevant information.

By reading this book, you understand that the writers, publishers, and any contributors engaged in the development of this material are not responsible for any damages, injuries, or losses that may occur from the use of the information contained here.

Always prioritize your health and safety, and seek competent medical advice for any issues linked to diabetes or any other health condition.

Copyright © by Richard B. Peltier 2023. All right reserved.

Before this document is duplicated or reproduced in any manner, the publisher's consent must be gained.

Therefore, the content within can neither in nor full can the document be copied, scanned, faxed, or retained without approval from the publisher or creator.

Table of Content

Introduction

Balancing Blood Sugar through Smart Nutrition

Welcome to "Balancing Blood Sugar: A Comprehensive Guide to Diabetes Meal Planning and Nutritious Eating." This book is your compass for navigating the world of diabetes control via smart meal planning and nutritious eating. Whether you're new to the domain of diabetes or trying to increase your current knowledge, this book is here to empower you with practical insights and efficient ways to attain stable blood sugar levels while relishing tasty and healthy meals.

Diabetes is a complicated illness that involves careful attention to numerous parts of your lifestyle, with diet being a cornerstone. Making thoughtful decisions about the meals you eat is not only vital for regulating blood sugar levels but also for supporting general health and well-being. This book is your trusted companion, presenting you with a detailed guide to preparing balanced and diabetes-friendly meals that will keep you motivated, satiated, and in charge of your health.

In the chapters that follow, we'll dig into the depths of diabetes, helping you grasp its nuances, causes, and the effect it has on your health.

We'll begin on a voyage of meal planning, studying the important components of a diabetes-conscious diet, and providing you with practical skills to make educated decisions in every culinary experience.

From interpreting food labels and portion control to navigating dining out and mastering mindful eating, we'll empower you with the information and skills to construct a well-rounded eating plan that corresponds with your diabetes management objectives. You'll discover a selection of healthful dishes, each intended to excite your taste buds while maintaining stable blood sugar levels.

However, please note that the material offered in this book has an instructional function. Diabetes management is very personalized, and talking with your healthcare professional or a qualified dietician is vital for adjusting the information to your particular requirements and circumstances. Your road towards balanced blood sugar and greater well-being begins here.

By learning to appreciate smart nutrition and creating a good connection with food, you're taking proactive steps towards a healthier and more vibrant existence.

Together, let's embrace the power of nutrition, make educated decisions, and go on a delightful journey that harmonizes your passion for food with your devotion to health.

Chapter 1

Understanding Diabetes

Diabetes is a chronic metabolic illness that affects millions of individuals worldwide. It happens when the body is unable to create enough insulin or efficiently use the insulin it produces. Insulin is a hormone generated by the pancreas that helps control blood sugar levels and enables glucose to enter the cells, supplying them with energy.

There are three primary forms of diabetes:

Type 1 Diabetes: Type 1 diabetes, also known as insulin-dependent diabetes or juvenile-onset diabetes, is an autoimmune disorder where the immune system erroneously assaults and kills the insulin-producing beta cells in the pancreas. As a consequence, people with Type 1 diabetes generate little or no insulin. This syndrome generally develops in infancy or adolescence and needs lifelong insulin treatment.

Type 2 Diabetes: Type 2 diabetes, previously known as adult-onset diabetes, is the most prevalent type of diabetes.

In this case, the body either doesn't create enough insulin or the cells develop resistance to insulin's actions, resulting in increased blood sugar levels. Several factors contribute to the development of Type 2 diabetes, including genetics, lifestyle choices, obesity, and physical inactivity.

Gestational Diabetes: Gestational diabetes arises during pregnancy and affects women who did not have diabetes before becoming pregnant. Hormonal changes during pregnancy may lead to insulin resistance, and if the pancreas cannot make enough insulin to compensate, it leads to gestational diabetes. While this illness normally disappears after delivery, women who have had gestational diabetes are at a greater risk of developing Type 2 diabetes later in life.

Causes and Risk Factors

The specific causes of diabetes are not entirely known; however, various variables contribute to its development.

Genetics: A family history of diabetes might raise an individual's chance of having the ailment. Certain genes may predispose someone to diabetes, making them more vulnerable.

Obesity and Sedentary Lifestyle: Excess body weight, particularly around the waist, is a substantial risk factor for Type 2 diabetes. Lack of physical exercise and a sedentary lifestyle may also contribute to insulin resistance.

Age: The risk of Type 2 diabetes rises with age, especially beyond the age of 45. However, owing to the increased frequency of paediatric obesity, Type 2 diabetes is increasingly affecting younger people as well.

Ethnicity: Certain ethnic groups, such as African Americans, Hispanics, Native Americans, and Asians, are at greater risk of acquiring diabetes compared to others.

Gestational Factors: Women who have had gestational diabetes in prior pregnancies or gave birth to big infants (over 9 pounds) are more likely to acquire Type 2 diabetes later in life.

Other Medical problems: Certain medical problems, such as polycystic ovarian syndrome (PCOS) and high blood pressure, might raise the risk of diabetes.

Symptoms and Complications

The symptoms of diabetes might vary based on the kind and severity of the ailment. Some typical symptoms include:

- Excessive thirst and hunger
- Frequent urination
- Fatigue and weakness;
- Unexplained weight loss;
- Blurred vision; Slow-healing wounds
- And frequent infections.

If left untreated or inadequately managed, diabetes may lead to significant complications that affect many organs and systems in the body, including;

Cardiovascular complications: Elevated blood sugar levels may damage blood vessels and lead to atherosclerosis.

Nerve Damage (Neuropathy): High blood sugar levels may damage the nerves, resulting in symptoms such as numbness, tingling, and pain in the hands and feet. Diabetic neuropathy may also impact the digestive tract, producing issues with digestion and bowel motions.

Kidney Damage (Nephropathy):

Diabetes is one of the primary causes of kidney failure. High blood sugar levels may damage the tiny blood capillaries of the kidneys, decreasing their capacity to filter waste from the blood properly.

Eye Complications (Retinopathy): Diabetes may damage the blood vessels in the retina, resulting in diabetic retinopathy, which can cause vision loss or blindness if left untreated.

Foot Complications: Nerve damage and poor circulation in the feet may lead to foot ulcers and infections, occasionally leading to the need for amputation.

Skin disorders: People with diabetes are more prone to skin disorders such as bacterial and fungal infections.

Pregnancy difficulties: Gestational diabetes may lead to difficulties during pregnancy, including high birth weight, early delivery, and a higher chance of acquiring Type 2 diabetes later in life.

The Importance of Blood Sugar Management:

Proper blood sugar control is critical for those with diabetes to avoid complications and maintain a decent quality of life.

This entails obtaining and maintaining target blood sugar levels using a mix of medication, food, physical exercise, and lifestyle adjustments.

- For people with Type 1 diabetes, insulin treatment is vital for life, and they must closely check their blood sugar levels throughout the day.
  This may require many daily injections or the use of an insulin pump, which supplies insulin constantly.
- For patients with Type 2 diabetes, blood sugar control frequently starts with lifestyle modifications, such as adopting a balanced and nutritious diet and increasing physical activity. In certain circumstances, oral medicines or insulin injections may be administered to help regulate blood sugar levels.

In conclusion: recognizing diabetes is the first step in properly treating the illness and lowering the risk of complications. With the correct education, skills, and support, people with diabetes may lead productive lives and take responsibility for their health and well-being. The next chapters will go further into diabetic meal planning and healthy eating practices to help people maintain stable blood sugar levels and attain maximum health.

Chapter 2:

Diabetes Meal Planning Basics:

Managing diabetes successfully starts with making educated and conscientious eating choices. Proper meal planning has a crucial role in managing blood sugar levels and sustaining general health. This chapter will dig into the basic concepts of diabetic meal planning, including understanding the influence of various foods on blood sugar, adopting proper portion sizes, and utilizing techniques to construct balanced and healthy meals.

The Role of Diet in Diabetes Management: Diet is an important component of diabetes care since the foods we consume directly impact our blood sugar levels. When we eat, our bodies break down carbs into glucose, which is the major source of energy for our cells. Insulin, a hormone generated by the pancreas, is important for promoting the absorption of glucose into cells, where it may be utilized for energy.

In patients with diabetes, there is either a lack of insulin (Type 1 diabetes) or an impaired response to insulin (Type 2 diabetes). As a consequence, the control of blood sugar becomes more complicated, resulting in variations in glucose levels.

Understanding the influence of various foods on blood sugar is vital for planning a diabetes-friendly diet.

1. Carbohydrates: Carbohydrates have the most significant influence on blood sugar levels. They are quickly broken down into glucose, creating a high spike in blood sugar after meals. Carbohydrates are found in foods such as grains, fruits, vegetables, legumes, and dairy products.

2. Proteins: Proteins have a little influence on blood sugar levels. While they may induce the release of insulin, the impact is rather minimal compared to carbs. Protein-rich foods include meat, fish, poultry, eggs, tofu, and dairy products.

3. Fats: Fats have a minor influence on blood sugar levels. However, it's vital to pick good fats, such as those found in avocados, nuts, seeds, and olive oil, since they boost heart health and general well-being.

Glycaemic Index and Glycaemic Load:

The glycaemic index (GI) is a measure of how rapidly a carbohydrate-containing diet elevates blood sugar levels. Foods with a high GI induce a quick spike in blood glucose, whereas those with a low GI have a longer and more progressive impact.

Incorporating low-GI foods into meals may help stabilize blood sugar levels since they contribute to more sustained energy and lower the likelihood of spikes and crashes. Examples of low-GI foods include whole grains, legumes, non-starchy vegetables, and certain fruits like berries and apples.

The glycaemic load (GL) takes into consideration both the glycaemic index of a meal and its carbohydrate content per serving. It delivers a more realistic picture of a food's influence on blood sugar. Foods with a low glycaemic load have a reduced influence on blood sugar levels and are preferred in diabetic meal planning.

Portion Control and Meal Timing:

In addition to knowing the influence of various foods, portion management is vital for those with diabetes. Eating excessive amounts, even of low-GI meals, may still lead to considerable spikes in blood sugar levels. Controlling portion sizes helps avoid overeating and maintains more consistent blood glucose levels throughout the day.

Spacing meals and snacks equally throughout the day is also crucial for blood sugar regulation. Consistent mealtime helps manage insulin levels and avoids severe variations in blood glucose.

It's typically suggested to have three balanced meals and incorporate healthy snacks in between, if required, to prevent lengthy periods of fasting.

The Plate Method for Balanced Meals:

The plate technique is a basic and efficient strategy to construct balanced meals that encourage stable blood sugar levels. It entails dividing your plate into exact quantities for various meal groups:

1. **Vegetables**: Fill half of your plate with non-starchy veggies, including leafy greens, broccoli, cauliflower, peppers, and tomatoes. These are low in calories and carbs yet rich in important vitamins, minerals, and fibre.

2. **Proteins**: Allocate a quarter of your plate to lean protein sources, such as fish, poultry, tofu, lentils, or lean cuts of meat. Protein helps you feel full and satisfied while having a little influence on blood sugar.

3. **Carbohydrates**: The remaining quarter of your plate may be allocated for healthy carbohydrate sources such as whole grains (brown rice, quintal, whole wheat), starchy vegetables (sweet potatoes, maize, peas), and fruits. Focus on low-GI choices to avoid sudden rises in blood sugar.

4. **Healthy Fats**: While not specifically depicted on the plate, healthy fats should be provided in moderation.

Add a modest dose of avocado, almonds, seeds, or olive oil to your meals to improve heart health and enhance fullness.

Creating a Well-Balanced Meal Plan:

Designing a well-balanced diet plan is vital for those with diabetes to maintain consistent blood sugar levels, reach a healthy weight, and avoid complications. Here are some crucial points to consider while designing a diabetes-friendly food plan:

1. **Consult a Registered Dietician**: Seeking help from a licensed dietician who specializes in diabetic nutrition may be immensely useful. They can help you build a meal plan that suits your individual dietary requirements, tastes, and health objectives.

2. **Be Mindful of Carbohydrates**: Carbohydrate counting is a typical method used by people with diabetes to regulate blood sugar levels. Keeping note of the quantity of carbs ingested in each meal will assist in calculating optimal insulin dosing, if required.

3. **Choose whole Foods**: Opt for whole, unprocessed foods wherever feasible. Fresh fruits, vegetables, whole grains, lean meats, and healthy fats should form the cornerstone of your diet.

Processed meals generally have added sugars, harmful fats, and excessive amounts of salt, which may significantly affect blood sugar and overall health.

4. Experiment with Meal Scheduling: Some people with diabetes may benefit from alternate meal scheduling techniques, such as intermittent fasting or time-restricted eating. These treatments may enhance insulin sensitivity and aid in blood sugar management. However, it's vital to talk with a healthcare practitioner before making any changes to your eating regimen.

5. Stay Hydrated: Drinking lots of water throughout the day is vital for general health and diabetes control. Water helps wash out impurities, aids digestion, and may help avoid excessive hunger, which may contribute to overeating.

6. Moderate Alcohol Consumption: If you prefer to consume alcohol, do it in moderation. Alcohol may induce variations in blood sugar levels and may interact with certain diabetic medicines. Always drink alcohol with meals and with your healthcare professional to confirm it is safe for you.

7. Practice Mindful Eating: Mindful eating is giving full attention to the sensory experience of eating, including the taste, texture, and scent of food.

It may help avoid overeating, improve digestion, and boost the enjoyment gained from meals.

8. Be Consistent with Physical activity. Regular physical exercise is a crucial component of diabetes treatment. Exercise may help enhance insulin sensitivity, reduce blood sugar levels, and boost general well-being. Aim to combine workouts that improve flexibility with aerobic activity and strength training..

Conclusion: Understanding the fundamentals of diabetic meal planning is vital for efficiently controlling blood sugar levels and sustaining overall health. By choosing suitable food choices, regulating portion sizes, and adopting a balanced plate strategy, people with diabetes may establish a sustainable and healthy meal plan. Moreover, working with healthcare experts and licensed dieticians may provide tailored direction and assistance in designing a diet that suits individual requirements and lifestyle choices. Consistent meal planning, combined with regular physical exercise and medication control, can allow people with diabetes to have healthier and more rewarding lives while successfully managing their disease.

Chapter 3

Building a Healthy Diabetes-Friendly Diet

Creating a nutritious and diabetes-friendly diet is vital for efficiently controlling blood sugar levels, maintaining a healthy weight, and lowering the risk of complications. This chapter will dig into the fundamental components of a diabetes-friendly diet, concentrating on adding nutrient-dense foods, limiting carbohydrate consumption, and making intelligent food choices to improve overall well-being.

The Importance of Whole Foods and Nutrient-Dense Choices:

 A diabetes-friendly diet should largely consist of complete, nutrient-dense foods that provide critical vitamins, minerals, and fibre without triggering abrupt rises in blood sugar. Nutrient-dense foods are those that have a high concentration of nutrients compared to their calorie level. Some examples of nutrient-dense foods include:

1. Non-Starchy Vegetables: Leafy greens, broccoli, cauliflower, Brussels sprouts, bell peppers, cucumbers, and zucchini are rich in vitamins, minerals, and fibre while being low in calories and carbs.

2. Lean Proteins: Skinless chicken, fish, tofu, legumes (such as lentils, chickpeas, and black beans), and low-fat dairy products are good sources of protein without contributing to large blood sugar spikes.

3. Whole Grains: Whole grains like equinox, brown rice, oats, and barley include complex carbs and fibre, which help balance blood sugar levels and give lasting energy.

4. Healthy Fats: Avocados, nuts, seeds, and olive oil are sources of monounsaturated fats that promote heart health and create a sensation of fullness.

5. Fruits: Opt for fruits with lower glycaemic index values, such as berries, apples, pears, and citrus fruits, which have a softer influence on blood sugar.

6. Low-Fat Dairy: Choose low-fat or non-fat dairy products like Greek yogurt or skim milk to limit saturated fat consumption.

By prioritizing whole foods and nutrient-dense selections, people with diabetes may enjoy a broad range of tasty and fulfilling meals while keeping their blood sugar levels under control.

Foods to Include:

1. Veggies: Aim to fill half your plate with non-starchy veggies at each meal. Incorporate a diversity of colours and textures to guarantee a broad nutritional intake.

2. **Lean Proteins**: Include lean proteins in every meal to help balance blood sugar levels and induce fullness. Opt for grilled, baked, or broiled dishes instead of fried choices.

3. **Whole Grains**: Choose whole grains over processed grains whenever feasible. These grains are richer in fibre, which slows down the breakdown of carbs and helps maintain stable blood sugar levels.

4. **Healthy Fats**: Use tiny quantities of healthy fats in cooking and as salad dressings. These fats not only supply important nutrients but also aid in the absorption of fat-soluble vitamins.

5. **Fruits:** Enjoy fruits in moderation and prefer whole fruits over fruit juices to benefit from their fibre content, which delays the absorption of glucose into the circulation.

6. **Low-Fat Dairy**: Incorporate low-fat or non-fat dairy products into your diet to guarantee optimal calcium intake for bone health.

Foods to Limit:

1. Refined Sugars: Minimize the intake of foods and drinks rich in added sugars, such as sugary sodas, sweets, pastries, and sweetened cereals. 2. Processed Foods: Reduce the consumption of highly processed foods that are generally heavy in harmful fats, added sugars, and salt. Instead, aim for full, unprocessed meals.

3. Saturated Fats: Limit the intake of foods rich in saturated fats, such as fatty cuts of meat, full-fat dairy products, and tropical oils like coconut and palm oil.

4. Salt: Monitor your salt consumption to enhance heart health and avoid excessive blood pressure. Choose low-sodium or salt-free options wherever feasible.

5. Alcohol: If you prefer to drink alcohol, do it in moderation. Alcohol may induce variations in blood sugar levels and interfere with diabetic treatments.

Creating a Well-Balanced Meal Plan

To design a well-balanced meal plan that promotes diabetes control, consider the following tips:

1. Count Carbohydrates: If you are following a carbohydrate counting plan, measure your carbohydrate consumption to help regulate blood sugar levels and alter insulin doses appropriately.

2. Balance Meals: Use the plate technique (as taught in Chapter 2) to produce balanced meals that contain proper servings of vegetables, meats, and carbs.

3. Snack Smartly: Choose nutritious snacks that mix a source of protein or healthy fat with a modest quantity of carbs to manage blood sugar levels between meals.

4. Keep Hydrated: Drink lots of water throughout the day to stay hydrated and promote overall health. Water has no effect on blood sugar levels.

5. Limit Portion Sizes: Even when selecting nutrient-dense meals, portion control is vital for weight management and blood sugar homeostasis.

6. Be Mindful of Timing: Be consistent with meal and snack times to encourage improved blood sugar management and maximize insulin use.

7. Read Labels: Pay attention to product labels to uncover hidden sugars, extra fats, and excessive salt concentrations in packaged meals.

Healthy Eating Tips for Specific Situations:

1. Eating Out: When eating out, seek establishments that provide healthier alternatives and be cautious of portion sizes. Request sauces, dressings, and condiments on the side to manage your consumption.

2. Traveling: Plan ahead and carry healthy snacks and meals for travel. Bring non-perishable goods like nuts, seeds, whole fruit, and whole-grain crackers.

3. Social Gatherings: Practice portion control at social occasions and focus on enjoying the people rather than indulging in excessive quantities of food.

4. Managing Hypoglycaemia: Always keep a fast-acting supply of glucose or carbs available to treat low blood sugar episodes.

5. Stress Eating: To avoid using food as a coping mechanism, learn appropriate coping mechanisms for stress management, such as exercise, meditation, or rewarding hobbies.

Conclusion: Building a nutritious and diabetes-friendly diet is crucial to regulating blood sugar levels, maintaining a healthy weight, and improving overall well-being. By concentrating on nutrient-dense whole foods, managing carbohydrate consumption, and adopting intelligent food choices, people with diabetes may improve their health and increase their quality of life. Remember that individual nutritional needs may vary, and it's crucial to consult with a healthcare expert or registered dietician to develop a meal plan that suits your personal requirements and health objectives. Embrace the adventure of finding tasty and satisfying meals that support your diabetes control and contribute to a lively and meaningful existence.

Chapter 4

Carbohydrate Counting and Blood Sugar Control

Carbohydrate counting is a valuable tool for individuals with diabetes, particularly those using insulin therapies to manage blood sugar levels effectively. Understanding how different carbohydrates impact blood sugar and learning how to count and monitor carbohydrate intake can help individuals make informed food choices, optimize insulin dosages, and maintain stable glucose levels throughout the day.

Understanding Carbohydrates and Their Effects on Blood Sugar:

Carbohydrates are the primary macronutrient that has the most significant impact on blood sugar levels. When consumed, carbohydrates are broken down into glucose, causing blood sugar levels to rise. This response triggers the release of insulin, which allows glucose to enter the cells and be used for energy.

The rate at which carbohydrates affect blood sugar varies depending on the type of carbohydrate and how it is prepared or processed.

Carbohydrates can be broadly categorized as:

1. **Simple Carbohydrates:** These are sugars that quickly raise blood sugar levels. Examples include table sugar (sucrose), fructose (found in fruits), and lactose (found in milk and dairy products).
2. **Complex Carbohydrates:** These consist of long chains of sugars and have a slower effect on blood sugar levels. Complex carbohydrates are found in whole grains, legumes, and starchy vegetables.

Carbohydrate Counting Basics:

Carbohydrate counting involves tracking the total grams of carbohydrates consumed in a meal or snack. By knowing the amount of carbohydrates in the foods they eat, individuals with diabetes can adjust their insulin doses appropriately, matching the insulin to the amount of carbohydrates ingested.

The standard unit for measuring carbohydrates is the "gram" (g). On food labels, the total carbohydrate content is usually listed, making it easier to count carbohydrates in pre-packaged foods. For foods without nutrition labels, such as fruits and vegetables, online resources and mobile applications can provide approximate carbohydrate values.

Practical Tips for Carbohydrate Counting:

1.Learn Serving Sizes: Familiarize yourself with standard serving sizes for common carbohydrate-containing foods.

For example, one serving of carbohydrates is typically equal to 15 grams of carbohydrates.

2. Use Measuring Tools: When possible, use measuring cups, spoons, or a food scale to accurately measure portions and track carbohydrate intake.

3. Record Your Intake: Keeping a food journal or using a mobile app to track carbohydrate intake can help you monitor your eating habits and make adjustments as needed.

4. Be Mindful of Hidden Carbohydrates: Some foods may contain hidden carbohydrates, such as sauces, condiments, and processed foods. Read labels carefully to identify these hidden sources.

5. Understand Glycaemic Load: In addition to counting carbohydrates, consider the glycaemic load (GL) of foods. The glycaemic load takes into account both the glycaemic index and the carbohydrate content of a food, providing a more accurate reflection of its impact on blood sugar.

Adjusting Insulin Doses with Carbohydrate Counting:

The goal of carbohydrate counting is to match insulin doses with carbohydrate intake to maintain target blood sugar levels. The insulin-to-carbohydrate ratio (ICR) is a personalized calculation that healthcare professionals use to determine how much insulin is needed to cover a certain amount of carbohydrates.

For example, if a person's ICR is 1:10 (1 unit of insulin for every 10 grams of carbohydrates) and they plan to eat a meal with 45 grams of carbohydrates, they would need to administer 4.5 units of insulin to cover the carbohydrates in that meal.

It's essential to work closely with a healthcare provider or diabetes educator to determine your specific ICR and to adjust insulin doses based on blood sugar readings and activity levels.

Advanced Carbohydrate Counting Techniques:

While some individuals may prefer a simple carbohydrate counting approach, others may benefit from more advanced techniques:

1. Carbohydrate Partitioning: This involves dividing carbohydrates into multiple smaller meals or snacks throughout the day to promote better blood sugar control.

2. Insulin Pump Therapy: Insulin pumps allow for more precise insulin delivery, including the ability to set temporary basal rates or use bolus calculators that consider carbohydrate intake and blood sugar levels.

3. Continuous Glucose Monitoring (CGM): CGM systems provide real-time data on blood sugar levels, helping individuals make more informed decisions about insulin dosing and carbohydrate intake.

Conclusion: Carbohydrate counting is a valuable tool for individuals with diabetes to manage blood sugar levels effectively. By understanding how different carbohydrates impact blood sugar and learning how to count and monitor carbohydrate intake, individuals can make informed food choices and optimize insulin dosages. It's essential to work closely with healthcare professionals or diabetes educators to develop a personalized carbohydrate counting plan that meets individual needs and lifestyle preferences. With practice and consistency, carbohydrate counting becomes a valuable skill that empowers individuals with diabetes to take charge of their health and well-being.

Chapter 5

Meal Planning Strategies for Diabetes

Meal planning is an important element of diabetes treatment that includes carefully choosing and preparing meals to maintain stable blood sugar levels, attain a healthy weight, and enhance overall well-being. This chapter will cover several meal planning tactics and give practical recommendations to develop diabetes-friendly meals that are both nutritional and entertaining.

Sample Meal Plans for Different Calorie Needs:
Meal planning starts with estimating individual calorie requirements based on criteria such as age, gender, activity level, and weight control objectives. Here are example meal plans for three different calorie needs *(1,500, 1,800, and 2,200 calories per day)* to offer a rough concept of how meals might be structured:

1,500-Calorie Meal Plan:

• Breakfast: Scrambled eggs with spinach and cherry tomatoes, whole-grain bread, and a small apple.

• Lunch: Grilled chicken salad with mixed greens, cucumbers, and vinaigrette dressing;

• Snack: Carrot sticks with hummus.

• Dinner: Baked salmon with rice and steamed broccoli.

• Dessert: Greek yogurt with berries.

2. 1,800-Calorie Meal Plan:

• Breakfast: Oatmeal with sliced bananas and a sprinkling of cinnamon, combined with a cooked egg.

• Lunch: a turkey and avocado wrap with a whole-grain tortilla and a side of mixed fruit

• Snack: Almonds and a little orange.

• Dinner: Brown rice, broccoli, bell peppers, and tofu in a stir-fry.

• Dessert: Baked pear with a drizzle of honey and a sprinkling of walnuts.

2,200-Calorie Meal Plan:

• Breakfast: Whole-grain pancakes with Greek yogurt and fresh fruit.

• Lunch: Quanta salad with roasted veggies, chickpeas, and feta cheese.

• Snack: Cottage cheese with pineapple chunks

• Dinner: Grilled shrimp with sweet potato mash and a side of green beans.

• Dessert: Dark chocolate square with a handful of raspberries.

Creating Weekly Menus and Grocery Shopping Tips:

Planning meals for the week helps ensure that you have all the required items on hand, decreasing the likelihood of making impulsive and less nutritious choices. Follow these strategies to build weekly meals and make your grocery shopping more efficient:

1. **Prepare Ahead**: Take some time at the beginning of each week to prepare your meals and snacks. Create a meal that contains a range of items to prevent boredom.

2. **Make a Shopping List**: Based on your meal plan, develop a shopping list with all the items you'll need for the week. Stick to the list when shopping to prevent extra purchases.

3. **Shop the Perimeter**: In the grocery store, focus on the outside aisles where fresh vegetables, lean proteins, and dairy items are frequently placed. Limit excursions to the inner aisles, which include more processed and packaged items.

4. Check Labels: When buying packaged goods, check the labels carefully to find hidden sugars, bad fats, and excessive salt levels.

5. Buy in Bulk: Consider purchasing non-perishable products, such as whole grains, nuts, and seeds, in bulk to save money and avoid waste.

6. Stock Up on Frozen Foods: Frozen fruits, veggies, and lean meats are practical choices to keep on hand when fresh ones are not accessible.

7. Avoid Shopping Hungry: Shop after eating a meal or having a snack to prevent the temptation to purchase unhealthy items while hungry.

Meal Prepping for Busy Days:

Meal preparation may be a game-changer for folks with hectic schedules, as it enables you to prepare and portion meals in advance, saving time and encouraging healthier choices.

1. Choose a Prep Day: Designate a day each week for food preparation. Sundays are popular alternatives for many individuals.

2. Batch Cook: Prepare larger amounts of specific items, such as lean meats, healthy grains, and roasted veggies, to use in numerous meals throughout the week.

3. Use Containers: Invest in meal prep containers to portion and store your food neatly. This makes it easy to get a ready-to-eat dinner while you're on the run.

4. Prep Snacks Too: Cut up veggies, portion out almonds or trail mix, and prepare nutritious snacks to be easily accessible throughout the week.

5. Label and Date: Properly label and date your prepared meals to preserve freshness and prevent misunderstanding.

Dining Out and Making Healthier Choices:

Eating out doesn't have to wreck your diabetic meal plan. With a few smart decisions, you can enjoy restaurant meals while still controlling your blood sugar:

1. Review the Menu in Advance: Check the restaurant's menu online before you arrive to pick healthier alternatives in advance.

2. Control Portion Sizes: Ask for smaller servings or try sharing an entrée with a buddy to minimize your carbohydrate consumption.

3. Customize Your Order: Don't hesitate to request alterations to suit your dietary demands. Ask for dressings and sauces on the side to limit their quantity.

4. Choose Grilled or Baked: Opt for grilled, baked, or broiled alternatives instead of fried or sautéed items.

5. Avoid Sugary Beverages: Stick to water, unsweetened tea, or liquids sweetened with artificial sweeteners.

Conclusion: Effective meal planning is a cornerstone of diabetes care that helps patients maintain stable blood sugar levels, attain a healthy weight, and improve overall well-being. By developing weekly menus, buying carefully, meal prepping for busy days, and making better choices while dining out, people with diabetes may enjoy a diverse and healthy diet that complements their health objectives. Flexibility and consistency in meal planning are vital, allowing for individualized options and flexibility for diverse conditions. Working closely with a healthcare physician or registered dietician may give further direction and support, ensuring that your meal plan is suited to your individual dietary requirements and tastes. Embrace the chance to experience tasty and gratifying meals while taking ownership of your diabetes care path.

Chapter 6

The Role of Physical Activity in Diabetes Management

Physical exercise is a strong tool for those with diabetes, giving multiple advantages for blood sugar control, cardiovascular health, weight management, and general well-being. This chapter covers the critical role of exercise in diabetes care, gives practical ideas for integrating physical activity into everyday living, and describes how various forms of exercise may favourably affect blood sugar levels.

Benefits of Physical Activity for Diabetes:

Regular physical exercise provides a range of advantages for those with diabetes:

1. Blood Sugar Control: Exercise helps reduce blood sugar levels by boosting the absorption of glucose into cells, even in the absence of insulin. It enhances insulin sensitivity, making the body more effective at utilizing the insulin it generates.

2. Weight Management: Engaging in regular physical exercise may aid with weight reduction or weight management,

Which is advantageous for those with Type 2 diabetes since excess weight can lead to insulin resistance.

3. Cardiovascular Health: Exercise strengthens the heart and cardiovascular system, lowering the risk of heart disease, hypertension, and stroke—conditions that individuals with diabetes are more prone to acquiring.

4. Blood Pressure Management: Physical exercise may help decrease blood pressure, which is vital for those with diabetes since high blood pressure can worsen issues.

5. Stress Reduction: Regular exercise may lower stress levels and enhance mood, leading to improved overall mental health.

6. Improved Lipid Profile: Exercise may boost "good" HDL cholesterol levels while reducing "bad" LDL cholesterol levels and triglycerides.

7. Increased Energy Levels: Engaging in physical exercise raises energy levels and lowers weariness, supporting a more active and vibrant lifestyle.

Types of Exercise for Diabetes:

Different forms of exercise may have varied impacts on blood sugar levels. A well-rounded exercise plan often includes a combination of aerobic workouts, strength training, and flexibility exercises.

1. Aerobic Exercise: Also known as cardio, aerobic workouts include activities that boost your heart rate and respiration, such as brisk walking, running, cycling, swimming, dancing, and aerobic courses. These exercises may enhance insulin sensitivity and aid in blood sugar management.

2. Strength Training: Resistance activities, such as weight lifting or utilizing resistance bands, help develop muscle mass and enhance metabolism. More muscle mass promotes greater glucose utilization and higher insulin sensitivity.

3. Flexibility Exercises: Stretching and flexibility exercises assist in increasing joint mobility and lowering the risk of accidents. Activities like yoga and Pilates may help promote relaxation and stress reduction.

Safe Exercise Guidelines for Diabetes:

While exercise delivers considerable advantages for diabetes control, it's crucial to exercise carefully to minimize possible problems. Here are some recommendations to follow:

1. Consult Your Healthcare Provider: Before beginning any fitness program, visit your healthcare practitioner to confirm it is safe for your unique health condition and to identify any special activity limits.

2. Start Slowly: If you are new to exercising or haven't been active for a long time, begin with low-impact exercises and gradually build intensity and duration.

3. Monitor Blood Sugar Levels: Check your blood sugar levels before, during, and after exercise, particularly if you take insulin or certain drugs that might induce low blood sugar (hypoglycaemia).

4. Remain Hydrated: Drink lots of water before, during, and after exercise to remain hydrated.

5. Carry a Snack: Have a fast-acting supply of glucose, such as glucose pills or juice, immediately accessible in case of hypoglycaemia.

6. Wear Appropriate Footwear: Choose supportive and well-fitted footwear to safeguard your feet, especially if you have diabetes-related neuropathy.

7. Warm-Up and Cool-Down: Always start with a warm-up and conclude with a cool-down to progressively raise and decrease your heart rate and limit the chance of injury.

Incorporating Exercise Into Daily Life:

Finding methods to include physical activity into your everyday routine may make exercise more sustainable and enjoyable.

1. Take Active Breaks: Stand up and walk about for a few minutes every hour, particularly if you have sedentary work.

2. Use the steps: Opt for steps instead of elevators or escalators wherever feasible.

3. Walk or Bike: Choose walking or cycling for short journeys instead of driving.

4. Gardening: Gardening is a wonderful way to keep active and interact with nature.

5. Play with Pets: Engage in active play with your pets, such as taking them for a walk or playing fetch.

6. Dance: Put on some music and dance around your living room for a fun and efficient exercise.

7. Join a Group: Consider joining a fitness class, sports club, or walking group for social connection and inspiration.

Setting Realistic Exercise Goals:

Set practical and realistic workout objectives that suit your fitness level and lifestyle. Gradually increase the intensity, length, and frequency of your exercises as you get more comfortable with exercising. Aim for at least 150 minutes of moderate-intensity aerobic activity or 75 minutes of vigorous-intensity aerobic activity each week, spaced out over at least three days, and add strength training activities at least two days per week.

Conclusion: Physical exercise is a strong tool for those with diabetes, giving multiple advantages for blood sugar control, cardiovascular health, weight management, and general well-being. By including a variety of workouts into your routine, monitoring blood sugar levels, and exercising safely, you may have a more active and rewarding life while successfully managing your diabetes. Set reasonable objectives, be persistent, and remember that every step towards a more active lifestyle is a step towards improved health.

Always with your healthcare physician before beginning any new fitness program to ensure it corresponds with your unique health requirements and circumstances. Embrace the pleasure and empowerment that regular physical exercise may offer to your diabetes control journey.

Chapter 7

Diabetes Self-Care and Emotional Well-Being

Living with diabetes involves continual self-care and control, not just in terms of physical health but also mental well-being. This chapter covers the significance of self-care practices in diabetes management, discusses the emotional elements of living with diabetes, and includes suggestions for maintaining a good perspective and mental resilience.

The Importance of Diabetes Self-Care:

Diabetes self-care entails actively managing many facets of the illness to attain maximum health and avoid complications. Key components of diabetic self-care include:

1. Blood Sugar Monitoring: Regularly measuring blood sugar levels helps patients make educated decisions regarding insulin doses, prescription modifications, and lifestyle choices.

2. Medication Management: Taking diabetic medicines as recommended and sticking to treatment programs is critical for maintaining stable blood sugar levels.

3. Healthy Eating: Following a balanced and diabetes-friendly diet, as outlined in earlier chapters, is vital for regulating blood sugar levels and general health.

4. Physical Activity: Engaging in regular exercise helps increase insulin sensitivity, improves weight control, and contributes to improved cardiovascular health.

5. Stress Management: High amounts of stress might alter blood sugar levels. Finding appropriate stress management strategies is crucial for diabetes treatment.

6. Foot Care: Regular foot exams and adequate foot care are necessary for those with diabetes since they are at a greater risk of foot-related problems.

7. Regular Check-ups: Attend planned visits with healthcare specialists for diabetes testing and preventative care.

Emotional Impact of Diabetes:

Living with diabetes may have a substantial emotional effect since it needs on-going attention and lifestyle modifications. Some frequent emotional issues addressed by people with diabetes include:

1. Stress and concern: Managing blood sugar levels, medicines, and food may be difficult, leading to concern about possible problems.

2. Depression: The burden of controlling diabetes may contribute to feelings of melancholy, pessimism, and depression.

3. Fear of Hypoglycaemia: Fear of low blood sugar episodes (hypoglycaemia) may induce some people to forgo essential medicine or insulin dosages.

4. Diabetes fatigue: Constantly managing diabetes may be burdensome, leading to feelings of fatigue and dissatisfaction.

Strategies for Emotional Well-Being:

Maintaining emotional well-being is vital for optimal diabetes control. Here are some techniques to improve mental resilience and emotional health:

1. Seek Support: Connect with family, friends, or support groups to share experiences and get emotional support.

2. Educate Yourself: Knowledge about diabetes and its care may help alleviate worry and empower people to take control of their condition.

3. Practice Stress Management: Engage in stress-reducing activities such as mindfulness meditation, deep breathing exercises, yoga, or hobbies that provide pleasure and relaxation.

4. Talk to a Professional: If symptoms of worry, sadness, or diabetes burnout linger, try talking to a mental health professional or counsellor who specializes in diabetes-related emotional issues.

5. Create Realistic objectives: Break down diabetic self-care responsibilities into simple parts and create realistic objectives to prevent feeling overwhelmed.

6. Celebrate Progress: Acknowledge and celebrate your victories, no matter how modest they may appear.

Every significant step towards diabetic control is worth celebrating.

7. Mindful Eating: Pay attention to your eating patterns and emotional triggers, and practice mindful eating to create a healthy connection with food.

8. Engage in Physical Activity: Exercise is not only excellent for physical health but also for mental well-being, as it may increase mood and decrease stress.

9. Practice Gratitude: Keep a gratitude notebook to concentrate on the good parts of life and create a more hopeful view.

Coping with Diabetes-Related Challenges:

Living with diabetes may bring numerous problems, but having a proactive and optimistic mentality can make a major difference.

1. Diabetes-Related Setbacks: Diabetes care may not always go as anticipated. Learn from setbacks and utilize them as chances for development and advancement.

2. Dealing with Hypoglycaemia: To manage the fear of hypoglycaemia, engage with your healthcare practitioner to alter medication doses and practice blood sugar monitoring.

3. Avoiding Diabetes Burnout: To avoid burnout, emphasize self-care, establish boundaries, and take breaks from diabetes treatment when required.

4. Managing Diabetes in Social Settings: Communicate your requirements with friends and family to maintain a supportive atmosphere during social occasions.

Conclusion: Diabetes self-care covers both physical health and emotional well-being. By carefully monitoring blood sugar levels, maintaining a balanced diet, participating in regular physical exercise, and adopting stress management practices, people with diabetes may better control their disease and avoid complications. Additionally, treating the emotional burden of diabetes via support, education, and mental health interventions is crucial for overall well-being. Remember that living with diabetes is a process, and it's crucial to be patient and compassionate with yourself. Seek help from loved ones, healthcare experts, and diabetic support groups to navigate the difficulties and successes of diabetes management. Taking a proactive approach to both physical and mental self-care helps people with diabetes enjoy happy and vibrant lives while efficiently managing their disease.

Chapter 8

Preventing Diabetes Complications

Preventing diabetic complications is an important element of diabetes care. While diabetes demands meticulous self-care, carefully regulating blood sugar levels and maintaining a healthy lifestyle may dramatically lower the risk of long-term problems. This chapter discusses typical diabetes-related issues, the significance of prevention, and ways to safeguard general health and well-being.

Understanding Diabetes Complications: Uncontrolled diabetes may lead to many consequences that affect different regions of the body. Some common diabetes-related problems include:

1. Cardiovascular Complications: Diabetes raises the risk of heart disease, heart attacks, strokes, and high blood pressure owing to the effect of high blood sugar on blood vessels and the heart.

2. Neuropathy: Elevated blood sugar levels may damage nerves, resulting in diabetic neuropathy. This illness may cause discomfort, tingling, numbness, and diminished feeling in the hands and feet.

3. Nephropathy: Diabetes may damage the kidneys, resulting to diabetic nephropathy, which can culminate in kidney failure.

4. Retinopathy: Elevated blood sugar levels may damage blood vessels in the retina, resulting in diabetic retinopathy and possibly causing vision loss or blindness.

5. Foot Complications: Diabetes-related nerve damage and poor circulation may lead to foot ulcers, infections, and, in extreme situations, amputation.

6. Skin Complications: Diabetes may lead to skin disorders such as bacterial and fungal infections, slow-healing wounds, and dry, itchy skin.

Importance of Preventing Complications:

Preventing diabetic complications is critical for preserving quality of life and minimizing healthcare expenses associated with treating complications. By proactively treating diabetes, people may dramatically minimize the chance of acquiring these problems and preserve better overall health.

Strategies for Preventing Diabetes Complications:

1. Blood Sugar Control: Keeping blood sugar levels within a target range,

as indicated by healthcare specialists, is critical for avoiding diabetic complications. Regular blood sugar monitoring, medication, adherence, and lifestyle modifications lead to improved blood sugar control.

2. Healthy Eating: Following a balanced and diabetes-friendly diet, as covered in earlier chapters, is vital for regulating blood sugar levels and minimizing problems.

3. Regular Physical Activity: Engaging in regular exercise helps increase insulin sensitivity, improves weight control, and enhances cardiovascular health, lowering the risk of problems.

4. Blood Pressure Management: Keeping blood pressure within a reasonable range is vital for avoiding cardiovascular problems. Lifestyle adjustments, medication, and frequent check-ups are necessary for regulating blood pressure.

5. Cholesterol Management: Monitoring and regulating cholesterol levels via diet, exercise, and medication, if required, may help lower the risk of cardiovascular issues.

6. Regular Check-ups: Attend planned visits with healthcare professionals for diabetes tests and preventative care.

Regular eye checks, foot exams, and kidney function testing are critical for early diagnosis and management.

7. Smoking Cessation: If you smoke, stopping is vital for minimizing the risk of diabetes-related cardiovascular problems.

8. Foot Care: Practicing frequent foot inspections and adequate foot care helps avoid foot-related issues, particularly if you have diabetes-related neuropathy.

9. Stress Management: Managing stress correctly is vital for general well-being and blood sugar regulation. Stress reduction approaches, such as mindfulness meditation and relaxation exercises, may be useful.

Educating and Empowering Yourself:

Understanding the significance of diabetes control and the possible dangers of complications allows people to take proactive efforts to preserve their health. Educate yourself on diabetes, its complications, and preventative efforts to make educated choices and actively engage in your treatment.

Conclusion: Preventing diabetic complications is a primary issue for those living with diabetes.

By maintaining adequate blood sugar management, adopting a healthy lifestyle, and attending frequent check-ups,

People may dramatically lower the risk of long-term issues. Recognize that diabetes control is a lifetime process that takes commitment and effort. Embrace the assistance of healthcare professionals, diabetes educators, and loved ones as you navigate this path. Taking responsibility for your diabetes care and adopting preventative tactics may lead to a better and happier life while lowering the risk of diabetes-related complications. Remember that the work you put into avoiding difficulties now will pay off in greater health and well-being in the future.

Chapter 9

Coping with Diabetes-Related Challenges

Living with diabetes poses different obstacles that might impair physical health, mental well-being, and general quality of life. This chapter addresses typical diabetes-related issues and presents techniques to deal with them successfully, promoting resilience and enhancing diabetes management.

Common Diabetes-Related Challenges:

1. Blood Sugar Fluctuations: Blood sugar levels may be unpredictable, leading to emotions of frustration and concern about maintaining control.

2. Dietary Restrictions: Following a diabetes-friendly diet may entail major modifications to eating patterns, which may be problematic for some people.

3. Medication Management: Keeping track of medicines, insulin injections, and blood sugar monitoring might seem stressful, leading to medication mistakes or missing doses.

4. Social and Family Pressures: Navigating social events, family gatherings, and dining out may be tough owing to worries about food choices and blood sugar control.

5. Dread of Complications: The dread of diabetes-related complications may create anxiety and tension, hurting mental well-being.

6. Diabetes Burnout: The continual treatment necessary for diabetes may contribute to feelings of burnout and exhaustion.

7. Financial Burden: The expense of diabetes supplies, prescriptions, and treatment may be financially onerous.

Strategies for Coping with Diabetes-Related Challenges:

1. Education and Knowledge: Educate yourself on diabetes management, complications, and self-care. Knowledge helps you make educated choices and lowers your fear of the unknown.

2. Seek Support: Connect with support groups or diabetic communities where you may share experiences, acquire insights, and get emotional support.

3. Effective Communication: Communicate your wants and concerns with healthcare providers, family members and friends to establish a support network that understands your issues.

4. Stress Management: Practice stress reduction strategies such as deep breathing, meditation, yoga, or participating in hobbies to manage stress and promote emotional well-being.

5. Mindfulness: Be present in the moment and practice mindful eating to establish a healthy connection with food and minimize emotional eating.

6. Positive Self-Talk: Replace negative ideas with positive affirmations to improve self-confidence and resilience.

7. Set Realistic objectives: Set attainable objectives for diabetes control and appreciate your victories, no matter how modest.

8. Create a pattern: Establish a daily pattern that involves blood sugar monitoring, medication management, exercise, and self-care activities to establish consistency and decrease feelings of overburden.

9. Diabetic Technology: Consider employing diabetic technology, such as continuous glucose monitoring (CGM) devices and insulin pumps, to simplify diabetes care and obtain greater insights into blood sugar patterns.

10. Professional Support: Reach out to diabetes educators, therapists, or mental health specialists with expertise in diabetes care for help and coping skills.

Dealing with Diabetes-Related Stress:

Living with diabetes may be stressful; however adopting appropriate coping methods helps lessen its impact:

1. Identify stresses: Identify particular stresses connected to diabetes management and establish solutions to alleviate them.

2. Exercise Regularly: Physical exercise is a wonderful way to relieve stress and enhance general well-being.

3. Practice Relaxation methods: Incorporate relaxation methods into your everyday routine, such as meditation or deep breathing exercises.

4. Prioritize Self-Care: Make time for things you like and prioritize self-care to rejuvenate physically and emotionally.

5. Accept Imperfection: Acknowledge that diabetes management may have its ups and downs, and it's good to have periodic setbacks.

Conclusion: Coping with diabetes-related issues needs a mix of education, perseverance, and a support network. By addressing the physical and emotional components of diabetes treatment, people may enhance their quality of life and establish effective coping skills. Recognize that it's natural to endure problems, but with effort and a positive outlook, you can conquer them and flourish with diabetes. Embrace the learning experience and the ability to develop and adapt as you manage your diabetes. Remember that you are not alone—reach out for assistance, discuss your requirements, and empower yourself to live a happy life while properly managing your diabetes.

Chapter 10

Living a Full and Healthy Life with Diabetes

Living with diabetes doesn't mean you can't have a full and healthy life. This chapter stresses the significance of developing a positive mentality, choosing lifestyle choices that promote overall health, and taking responsibility of your diabetes management to lead a meaningful life.

Embracing a Positive Mind-set:

A positive outlook is a valuable aid in diabetes treatment. It may enhance your emotional well-being, build resilience, and drive you to make healthy choices.

Here are some strategies to create a happy outlook:

1. Gratitude Practice: Regularly express thanks for the wonderful elements of your life and diabetes experience. Focus on the potential for development and learning.

2. Mindfulness: Be present in the moment and practice mindfulness to decrease stress and boost appreciation for life's small joys.

3. Positive Self-Talk: Replace self-criticism with self-compassion. Encourage yourself, recognize victories, and understand that controlling diabetes is a constant learning process.

4. Set Realistic objectives: Establish attainable objectives for your diabetes control and celebrate achievement, no matter how modest.

5. Celebrate Achievements: Acknowledge your achievements in controlling diabetes, conquering hurdles, and preserving general health.

Making Healthy Lifestyle Choices:

Lifestyle choices have a key role in diabetes control and general well-being. By adopting healthy practices, you may maximize your health and decrease the chance of complications.

Balanced Diet:

1. Follow a balanced and diabetes-friendly diet, as outlined in earlier chapters, to support blood sugar management and general health.

2. Regular Exercise: Engage in regular physical exercise that you love to increase insulin sensitivity, control weight, and promote cardiovascular health.

3. Adequate Sleep: Prioritize adequate sleep, as it plays a critical role in blood sugar management, hormone balance, and general wellness.

4. Stress Management: Practice stress reduction strategies to lessen the effect of stress on blood sugar levels and mental well-being.

5. Avoid Smoking and Limit Alcohol: Quit smoking to lower cardiovascular risks and limit alcohol use, since it might impair blood sugar regulation.

Building a Support Network:

Surrounding oneself with a supportive network may make a huge difference in controlling diabetes and keeping a good outlook.

1. Family and Friends: Share your diabetes journey with loved ones and enable them to support and encourage you.

2. Diabetes Educators and Healthcare Providers: Work closely with diabetes educators and healthcare experts to obtain assistance and keep up-to-date with diabetes management.

3. Diabetic Support Groups: Join local or online diabetic support groups to connect with people having similar issues, share experiences, and exchange information.

Taking Charge of Diabetes Management:

Empower yourself to take an active part in your diabetes management:

1. Knowledge is Power: Stay updated on diabetes, its care, and the newest breakthroughs in treatment and technology.

2. Regular Check-ups: Attend regular check-ups with healthcare experts to monitor your diabetes, discover any concerns, and make appropriate modifications.

3. Blood Sugar testing: Stay consistent with blood sugar testing to learn how various circumstances impact your levels and make educated choices.

4. Advocate for Yourself: Communicate with healthcare professionals, voice your concerns, and actively engage in your care choices.

5. Continuous Learning: Be open to learning and adapting to new tactics and technology that might increase your diabetes care.

Finding Joy in Life:

Living a complete life with diabetes entails finding joy and following your passions:

1. Engage in Hobbies: Dedicate time to hobbies and activities that offer you pleasure and relaxation.

2. Traveling: With adequate planning and preparation, traveling is doable with diabetes. Explore new regions and cultures, but ensure you have adequate supplies and assistance.

3. Enjoy Social Activities: Participate in social events and gatherings with family and friends, concentrating on connections and joyful moments.

Conclusion: Living a full and healthy life with diabetes is within grasp. By establishing a positive mentality, adopting good lifestyle choices, creating a support network, taking an active part in diabetes management, and finding pleasure in life's events, you may flourish with diabetes. Remember that diabetes control is a constant process, and it's good to have ups and downs. Embrace the learning process, be patient with yourself, and appreciate the improvements you make along the way. With drive, perseverance, and a positive attitude, you may enjoy a meaningful life while efficiently controlling your diabetes.

Chapter 11

Overcoming Diabetes Management Challenges

Managing diabetes comes with its own unique set of challenges, and it's essential to equip yourself with strategies to overcome them effectively. This chapter addresses common obstacles faced by individuals with diabetes and provides practical solutions to tackle them.

1. Managing Blood Sugar Fluctuations:

• Regularly monitor blood sugar levels to understand patterns and identify potential triggers.

• Work with your healthcare provider to adjust medication doses or insulin regimens as needed.

• Keep a record of food intake, exercise, and stress levels to pinpoint factors affecting blood sugar levels.

• Learn to recognize and treat hypoglycaemia and hyperglycaemia promptly.

2. Dealing with Diabetes Burnout:

• Take breaks when needed and ask for support from loved ones or a diabetes support group.

• Set achievable diabetes management goals to avoid feeling overwhelmed.

• Focus on small successes and celebrate progress to stay motivated.

• Consider using diabetes management apps or technology to simplify daily tasks.

3. Handling Social and Family Pressures:

• Communicate your needs and boundaries to family and friends regarding diabetes management.

• Educate them about diabetes to foster understanding and support.

• Plan ahead for social gatherings to ensure diabetes-friendly food options.

• Engage in open discussions about diabetes to address concerns and misconceptions.

4. Coping with Diabetes-Related Anxiety:

• Practice relaxation techniques, such as deep breathing or meditation, to reduce anxiety.

• Seek counselling or therapy to address underlying fears and concerns.

• Join a diabetes support group to connect with others facing similar challenges.

• Engage in physical activity to release endorphins and improve mood.

5. Addressing Financial Challenges:

• Explore cost-saving options for diabetes supplies, such as buying in bulk or using patient assistance programs.

• Discuss medication cost concerns with your healthcare provider to explore more affordable alternatives.

• Seek information about insurance coverage and potential financial assistance programs for diabetes management.

6. Improving Medication Adherence:

• Use medication reminders, alarms, or smartphone apps to stay on track with medications.

• Keep medications in a visible and easily accessible place to avoid forgetting doses.

• Establish a daily routine that incorporates medication management.

• Educate yourself about the importance of medication adherence in diabetes management.

7. Navigating Diabetes and Exercise:

• Consult your healthcare provider before starting any exercise regimen, especially if you have complications or other health conditions.

• Choose physical activities you enjoy to increase motivation and adherence.

• Monitor blood sugar levels before, during, and after exercise to adjust your routine as needed.

• Engage in a variety of exercises, including aerobic, strength training, and flexibility activities, for overall health benefits.

8. Handling Stress and Diabetes:

• Identify stress triggers and implement stress-reduction techniques, such as yoga, meditation, or spending time in nature.

• Incorporate hobbies or activities that bring joy and relaxation into your daily routine.

• Seek support from loved ones, friends, or a mental health professional to cope with stress.

Conclusion:

Living with diabetes requires navigating various challenges, but with determination and proactive strategies, you can overcome them effectively. By focusing on blood sugar control, addressing emotional well-being, seeking support, and making lifestyle adjustments, you can enhance your diabetes management and improve your overall quality of life.

Remember that you are not alone in your diabetes journey—reach out to your healthcare team, loved ones, or diabetes support groups for guidance and encouragement. Embrace the learning process and celebrate the progress you make as you manage diabetes with resilience and determination.

Conclusion

Living Well with Diabetes

Managing diabetes is a journey that involves effort, education, and perseverance. Throughout this thorough guide, we have studied numerous elements of diabetes, from understanding the illness and its varieties to learning about good nutrition, physical exercise, and preventing complications. The key to living well with diabetes comes from empowering yourself with information, making educated decisions, and having a positive outlook.

As you begin your diabetes control journey, know that you are not alone. Your healthcare team, including physicians, diabetes educators, and support groups, is available to guide and assist you every step of the way. Building a solid support network with family and friends may also be beneficial in addressing the difficulties of diabetes together.

Take responsibility of your diabetes care by frequently checking your blood sugar levels, sticking to recommended medicines, and adopting a balanced and diabetic-friendly diet. Engaging in regular physical exercise and having a healthy lifestyle are crucial components of successfully controlling diabetes and avoiding complications.

Recognize that diabetes control is not always simple, and it's normal to encounter setbacks. Embrace a positive outlook, enjoy your triumphs, and learn from your experiences to consistently improve your diabetes management abilities.

Always emphasize self-care, including appropriate sleep, stress reduction, and treating your emotional well-being. Managing diabetes is not only about statistics and treatments; it's about nourishing your entire health and quality of life. Remember that diabetes does not define you. You are more than your disease, and with appropriate care and support, you can have a full, vibrant, and rewarding life.

As medical science and technology continue to develop, new medicines and techniques for treating diabetes may emerge. Stay updated about the newest advancements and be open to adopting them into your diabetes care strategy when appropriate.

Above all, be gentle to yourself. Diabetes control may be hard, but you have the power and tenacity to conquer any hurdles that come your way.

Take one step at a time, remain devoted to your health, and enjoy the path of living well with diabetes. With determination, education, and a positive approach, you may flourish with diabetes and attain a life filled with excellent health and well-being.

9 7 9 8 8 5 8 3 7 0 6 9 7